Allergy and Intolerance:

A dietary response

By

Lynne D M Noble

Copyright 2024 Lynne D M Noble

Independently published

About the Author

Lynne Noble was born in 1953 in Huddersfield, West Yorkshire. From a very early age, Lynne showed an interest in nutrition and genetics avidly reading any books that she could get her hands on at the time.

Initially, Lynne studied orthopaedics but events led her to work with the elderly mentally infirm. Here, her interest in neurodegenerative disorders and pain syndromes developed.

Lynne undertook rigorous programmes of study, completing her Cert Ed., (FE) BSc (Hons) and Adv. Dip Education simultaneously before moving onto her M.Ed.

From there she took further demanding programmes in Human Nutrition, Pharmacology, Neuroscience, Genetics and Immunology. During this time, she was given many prestigious awards for her academic work. It was noted then that Lynne was not afraid of tackling difficult subjects.

She began her law degree but ill health prevented her from pursuing this. However, in this time, she moved from being a foster parent to adoptive parent.

She has been instrumental in setting up projects in the community for disadvantaged groups.

She is a member of the Guild of Health Writers.

Now retired, she lives in a picturesque village in West Yorkshire with her husband. She enjoys gardening, watching her husband bowling and researching.

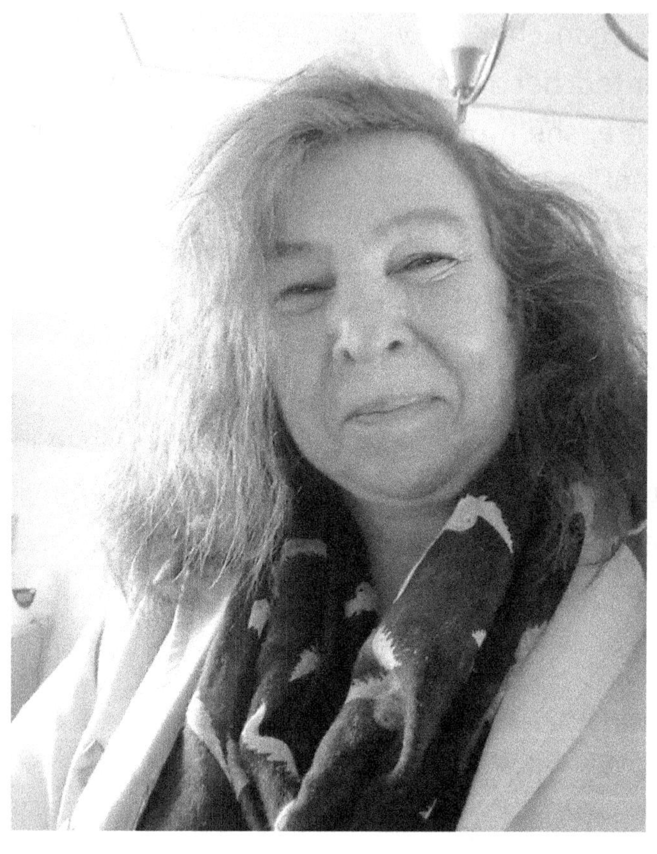

Author Lynne Noble at home

https://quintessentiallylynne.weebly.com/nutritional-medicine.html

contents

Introduction

Allergies, in all their forms, impact on lives in ways that we would not have imagined. Many children take important exams at the height of the hay fever season, children are driven to distraction by an itching, flaking rash known as eczema which does not seem to be controlled in spite of various medications. Asthma can impact on the ability to join in and enjoy sports unless it is well controlled.

Most people have heard of those unfortunates who have a peanut allergy. They may have even heard of something known of anaphylaxis but when I have mentioned 'angioedema' to them, their brows draw together as a look of puzzlement settles into their features. Then they will take a deep breath and say, 'Angie what?'

When I explain that it is swelling in the deeper layers of the skin, they cannot see what all the fuss is about until I explain that it can cause such swelling in the throat that it becomes life threatening. Any part of the body can swell including the gastrointestinal tract which creates a lot of discomfort for the sufferer. These unseen disabilities cause discomfort for the sufferer in more ways than one.

Angioedema isn't straightforward either. It can be underpinned by an allergic response but often no offending allergen can be found. In this case the angioedema is referred to as idiopathic which, in some ways, makes it more difficult to live with as you never know what is going to set it off and when. As such you can't avoid the 'trigger.'

I have come to the conclusion that 'idiopathic' angioedema is due to a real nutritional deficiency but no profit is to be made chasing up – and treating a nutritional deficiency; it's far easier to label it as 'idiopathic.'

This book looks at allergies in general and angioedema, although not all swelling can be attributed to angioedema even if there is a history of allergic type responses. However, more importantly, I investigate what the likely nutritional causes of angioedema type symptoms are and how these can be addressed.

The book is well illustrated since this helps to understand the impact of this condition on people's lives.

The difference between allergy and intolerance aids the beginning of understanding

People often use these terms as though they are interchangeable but they are not.

A proper allergic response involves an immunoglobulin (antibody) which is specific to allergy. It is immunoglobulin E and we write it as IgE in its short form.

There are other immunoglobulins which you may be familiar with. The two most common are IgG which will be raised in general infection and IgA which is raised in infections which attack the mucous membranes found in the respiratory system and the gastrointestinal tract.

When a reaction to a substance is a proper allergic reaction then it must involve an increase in IgE. This may occur due to substances which have been inhaled, touched or swallowed.

An allergic reaction is an over-reaction to substances that would not produce a reaction in the majority of the population.

While most reactions are mildly irritating – like the itchy rash you get if you walk through nettles – some are life- threatening and require the use of an Epipen.

It is far better to avoid the trigger and make sure that the diet is nutritionally sound. Sometimes you can find families where one child appears to be terribly afflicted and another doesn't where the difference had been made by diet.

In some cases, like that of my aunt, the propensity to angioedema will always have been there but her diet was sufficient to deal with and stave off any reaction. As she aged, and ate less well, the nutritional brakes disappeared and her angioedema appeared.

For some reason, peanut allergies appear to have become popular. I describe it like this as I never came across anyone with a peanut allergy when I was a child. It is not as if we didn't come into contact with it; post war, when food was scarce, saw a huge upsurge in the popularity of peanut butter to supply the protein and B vitamins that we required.

Nowadays, of course, they tend to be roasted in rapeseed oil. Some research undertaken by Fiocchi et al in 2016 found that rapeseed oil caused facial urticaria and abdominal discomfort.

Given that rapeseed oil is added to just about every processed food and ready meal, it is hard to avoid it.

We did not have this problem when our sources of fats were butter, lard and dripping.

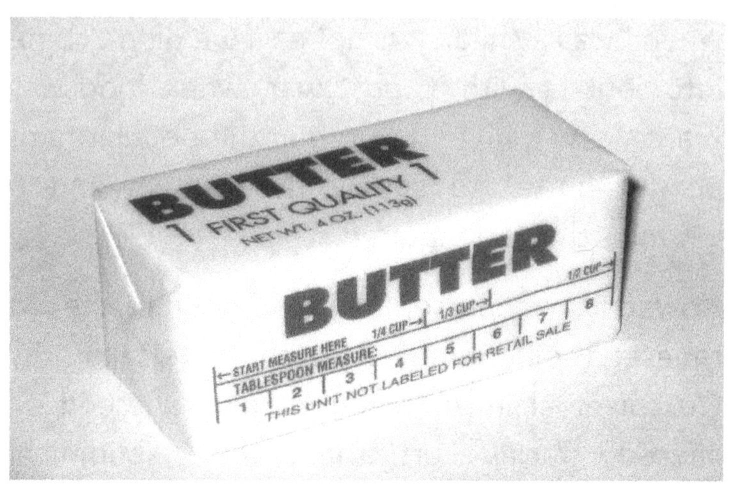

Butter does not cause allergic responses like rapeseed oil can do

By now you have probably gathered that a histamine intolerance or indeed, an intolerance of any kind, does not involve an IgE reaction. There is still a reaction; it is still unpleasant; it can be life threatening but it involves a different response which does not include IgE.

In order to determine if the reaction is an allergic one or an intolerance, then simple blood tests will be taken to look for the presence of antibodies.

A Personal Story

Like many people who suddenly find that they have a condition that nobody seems to know a great deal about, the responsibility for understanding it, falls mainly on us.

I started with symptoms of angioedema at the age of twenty- five. I didn't know what it was. My face swelled, my eyes closed up. I went to my GP more out of vanity, than anything. I was prescribed diuretics. I could understand this, in a way; there is kidney dysfunction in the family. However, this was found not to be the cause. Kidney problems have never affected me. At that time no further tests were undertaken. However, for some reason, I continued to be prescribed the diuretics. With hindsight, they probably exacaberated the condition. Many medications are a risk factor for angioedema but they are rarely given the attention they deserve. Indeed, many medics will say that, as the angioedema symptoms started before the medication was prescribed then the cause cannot possibly be the medication.

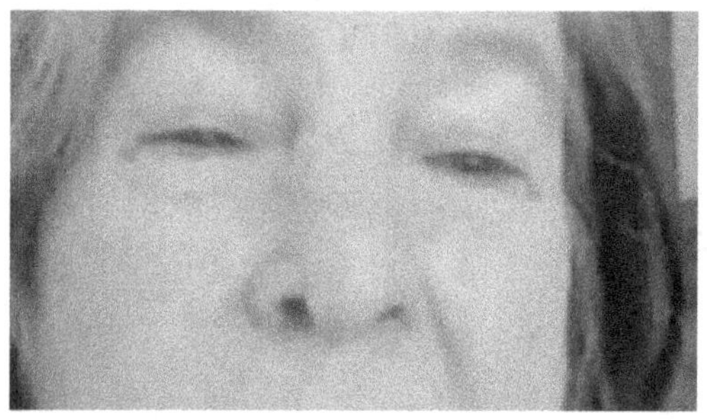

 Mild orbital swelling is quite common, on a daily basis with a condition like angieodema

I had a number of allergies such as hay fever, urticaria and asthma but nobody related the facial swelling to angieodema. I'd never heard of the medical condition, myself. Eventually, it was assumed that my symptoms were some sort of allergic reaction. However, this was decades down the line. By this time, the swelling also affected other parts of my body. It came, it went. There wasn't any pattern to it that I could ascertain. There wasn't any particular food that I could link it to, either.

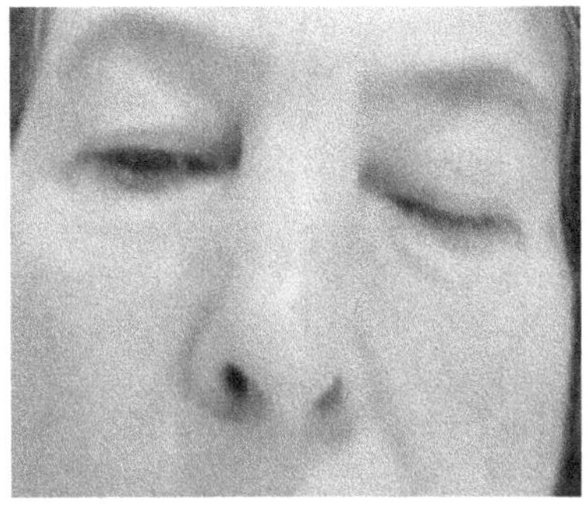

Facial flushing and orbital oedema

Eventually, I was referred to the immunology department. I was glad that the underlying reason was going to be established (I thought). By this time, my niece who was considerably younger was also experiencing similar symptoms. She sent me a photo of her hand which had swollen up in a matter of minutes. She hadn't injured it in any way. It was a mystery.

Just as mysteriously, it had disappeared after a few hours. She had not experienced pain at any time.

 It is amazing how angieodema can impact your life since the swelling can distort body parts in matters of seconds including facial features.

At the same time one of the younger relatives was posting up pictures of her hands swelling. My elderly aunt, who was in her 80's, developed what she was informed was urticaria but she likened it to deep itching that she couldn't eliminate. The fact that it was on her buttocks did not help as she could not help but scratch in order to try and alleviated the discomfort.

She wrote to me often speaking of how intolerable it was; not only because of the itching but the fact that in her 80's, the medical profession treated her as a non-entity. Once, having waited more than an hour past her appointment time, which is difficult at that age, she took herself and sat on the waiting room floor stating that she would not get up untll she was seen.   She was seen immediately and prescribed antihistamines in ever increasing doses.

The link of antihistamines   with dementia is well known and it was not the best treatment. However, it was the only one offered because the NHS is not allowed to look at this condition from a nutritional viewpoint.

Like my aunt I had mild allergic type symptoms; odd bouts of urticaria, cleaning materials made me sneeze; much to my disgust I had some food intolerances but I didn't let them spoil my lifestyle.

I didn't take antihistamines because they had a soporific effect and I didn't take kindly to feeling hung over all the time.

Eventually, I was referred to the immunology department.   I was glad that the underlying reason was going to be established (I thought). By this time, another niece who was considerably younger than I was,   was also experiencing similar symptoms. She sent me a photo of her hand which had swollen up in a matter of minutes.

She hadn't injured it in any way. It was a mystery.

My aunt wrote about that time, too. She had been taken off her usual antihistamines and was placed on high doses of Fenofexadine. It worked for about 12 hours and then the itching came back. She was prescribed twice the original dose.

She began to lose her memory a little. Histamine is required in the formation of memories and, of course, her antihistamines were blocking the histamine that she did need to help her keep alert.

External swelling is easy to see. It is easier to understand that when certain body parts are swollen that some loss of function will occur.

It is harder on everyone when the   lining of the gastrointestinal tract swells. It is one of those hidden disabilities even though the discomfort and pain is very real. It appears to run in the maternal side of the family; our reluctance to discuss any discomfort – as it just wasn't done to do so - made this information unknown to us until we were well past retirement age.

Just as facial and osesophageal swelling can be quite marked to the point it is life threatening, swelling to the lining of the gastrointestinal tract can also be profound. It's just that you can't see it but you can certainly feel the effects.

I had the usual range of tests but they did not reveal any allergic reaction. However, I was only tested for twenty of the most common allergens. There are literally hundreds of allergens so it was quite possible that I did have an allergy to something else that I hadn't been tested for.   Given that I had hay fever and mild asthma, the fact that nothing showed up an IgE reaction did not go down well with me.

After the tests were completed, I was informed that I had angioedema. It was explained that angioedema is a swelling of the lower layers beneath the skin, similar to urticaria or hives but the difference was that urticaria affects the upper layer of the skin while angioedema affects the deeper layers. This includes the:

- Dermis
- Subcutaneous tissue
- The mucosa
- Submucosal tissues

I was informed that I had 'idiopathic angioedema.

 This simply means that they do not know what the cause is. However, I also have:

- Cholinergic angioedema
- Physical angioedema

Cholinergic simply means that my tissues swell in response to heat. This was probably the worst part of this condition and I certainly did not enjoy summer.

Physical/exercise induced angioedema simply means that the swelling is induced by exercise.

I love walking but within a very short time, my ankles will have swollen a great deal. It takes a lot longer for the swelling to go than it does for the oedema to increase my foot size as much as it does.

It doesn't hurt but it is inconvenient –and expensive - when you need different sizes of shoes to accommodate the swelling.

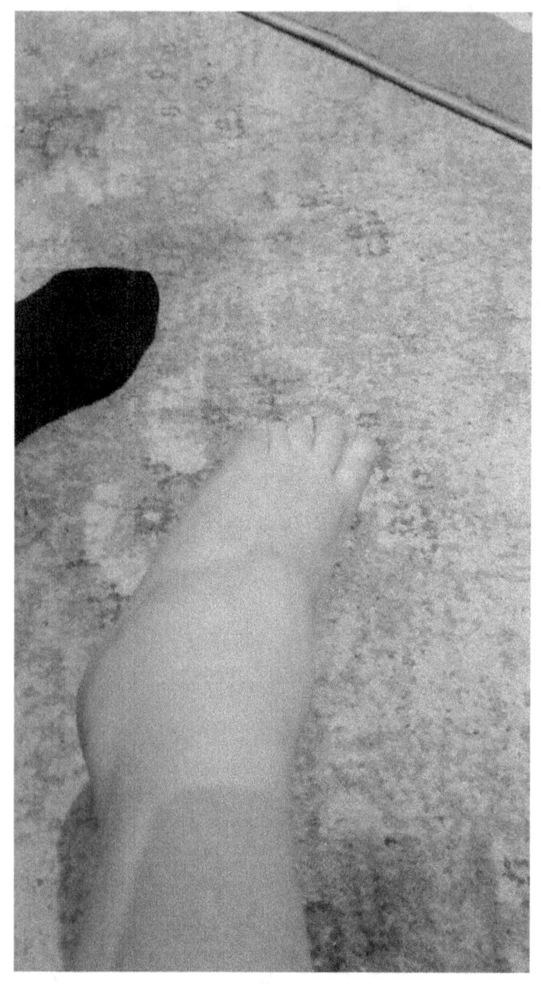

swelling occurs due to simple exercise

I did ask if it was familial but was assured that it was not. This was surprising since, as I have already stated, my aunt had also been diagnosed with angioedema. In her case, though, she was in her mid-80's, so why had this susceptibility been suppressed until then?

Although most of it occurred on her buttocks on one occasion, when I went to visit her and we went out for a meal, within minutes of eating one side of her lips had swollen up noticeably. When I remarked on it she informed me that it happened quite regularly.

 My niece still had periodic bouts of swelling and urticaria. She also had asthma and irritable bowel syndrome. Angieodema of the lining of the gastrointestinal tract will present as irritable bowel syndrome.

There are tests for hereditary angioedema and mine came back negative. I can only conclude that medicine needs to evolve more because more cases of angioedema, similar to my own, continued to turn up in the maternal side of the family. There certainly was a familial association even if it could not be ascertained. Perhaps there was some other familial trait not related to an actual allergy but, nevertheless, caused similar symptoms.

Before we can answer that, it is helpful to know what hereditary angioedema is.

Hereditary Angioedema

There are three main types of hereditary angioedema. The first two types are caused by a mutation in a gene that makes an inhibitor protein C1.

C1 inhibitors are a type of protein which help to moderate the body's inflammatory response. They act as a regulatory protein in part of the immune system known as the complement system which is a vital part of the innate immune system; this has a general defence function instead of the acquired immune system which has a more specialist function.

The third type of hereditary angioedema occurs due to gene mutation in factor XII. When this gene mutation occurs excessive amounts of bradykinin are produced. Bradykinin is a protein which induces inflammation. It causes blood vessels to dilate and this induces swelling. This occurs via the release of prostacyclin and nitric oxide among others.

As nitric oxide is intimately connected to nitrates then nitrates may be a culprit in angioedema in *some* individuals. Nitric oxide is linked with migraine headaches. My life was plagued by migraine headaches but, at that point - nor for many years later – did I make the connection.

Nitrates are chemicals that are found in the environment – in soil, water and air so they are ubiquitous. Nitrates may be added to food to stop the growth of bacteria. In addition, they also enhance the flavour of foods. Indeed, they are added to many foods to help preserve them. This is not good news for those who are predisposed to migraine headaches or angioedema.

Nitrates are also used in some medications. Their ability to dilate arteries is useful in conditions such as angina where the pain of angina is due to narrowed arteries. Unfortunately, common side effects of nitrates include:

- Flushing
- Headache
- Dizziness
- Low blood pressure
- Nausea
- swelling

The American Gut Project research has found that migraineurs have higher levels of bacteria which are normally involved in processing nitrates. Eventually, nitrates turn into nitric oxide which is associated with headaches.

Nitrates are found in many foods including:

- chocolate – especially dark chocolate and cocoa
- bacon
- wine
- processed meats in general
- beets
- garlic
- leafy green vegetables
- citrus fruits
- nuts and seeds

Normally, medics encourage patients to include these foods in their diet as they help to lower blood pressure. However, for migraineurs – or for those with nitrate induced angioedema - this isn't practical   given the impact on the sufferer's life.

It may be that some of the above foods impact, more than others, for the potential to cause migraine and angioedema. Most of the above, I have subconsciously avoided throughout my life, because they made me feel ill. However, I have never had a problem eating leafy green vegetables or beets, that I know of.

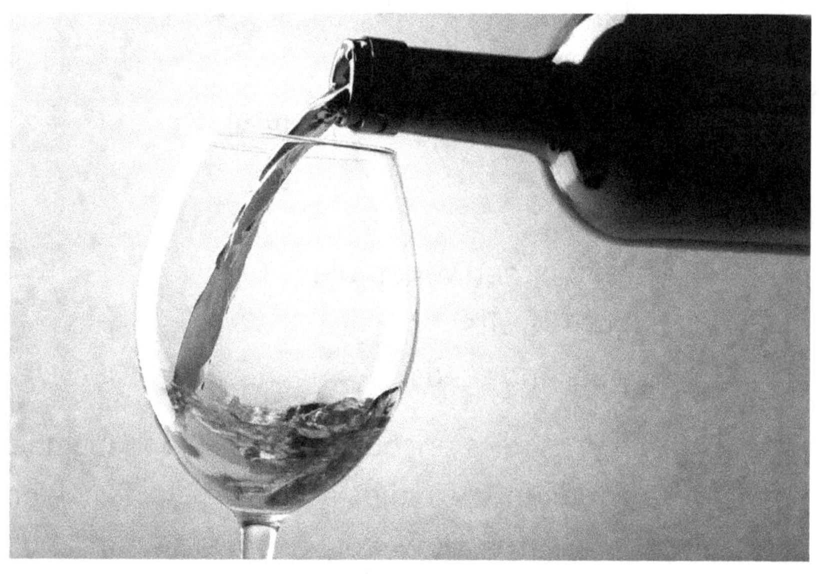

Red wine is well known for causing migraine

Hereditary angioedema is generally inherited from   a parent or parents in an **autosomal dominant** fashion.   This means that an abnormal gene from one person only can cause the disease.

Sometimes, it can occur *de novo* - as a new mutation - but, in my case, given the preponderance of this condition in the maternal side, this was unlikely.

Often there are triggers - other than food triggers. Minor trauma or stress can also induce bouts of angioedema.

Diagnosis of types I and II of these hereditary types is diagnosed through the measurement of C4 and C1 protein   inhibitor levels.

So, it was established that the cause of my angioedema was not due to insufficient C1 or C4 inhibitor levels nor was it due to a gene mutation on factor X II.

Fexofenadine is generally prescribed for angioedema. It is a large tablet and not available in liquid form. It is difficult to swallow if you have angioedema of the throat. However, it is gastric coated and therefore, it should not be broken up to make swallowing easier.

Sometimes Tranexamic acid is prescribed. Tranexamic acid is a medication used to treat or prevent excessive loss of blood from injury or post-partum haemorrhage, among others. It has also been found to be effective for hereditary angioedema, although it may take months before the effect is seen.

Tranexamic acid comes in a tablet form but this time the tablets are even larger than the Fexofenadine.

The beauty of Tranexamic acid if you are able to swallow it, is that side effects are rare.

Fexofenadine is a second generation H1-antihistamine. Second generation H1-antihistamines do not penetrate readily into the brain as the older first generation of antihistamines did. There, the first generation antihistamines cause drowsiness, fatigue and impaired concentration.

The impact on memory was detrimental to work performance of those taking them. It is not recommended that they are taken if driving or using machinery. In fact, it is recommended that first generation antihistamines are avoided altogether. However, they are quite effective against sleep disorders although a hang-over effect may occur the following day, after use.

Some of the first most popular first generation antihistamines are:

- Diphenydramine (Benadryl)
- Chlorphenamine (Tavist)

I was unable to continue taking Fexofenadine as it caused me to have flu like symptoms. Eventually, I tried a number of antihistamines that either came in liquid form or came in tablet form that was smaller and much easier to swallow. These included:

- Loratidine
- Cetirizine
- Piriton

Eventually, I settled on Cetirizine but turned out to be only a temporary measure. It was very small, easy to carry around and swallow and, it was for the most part, effective. It was also available over the counter at a very reasonable price. However, it had marked sedating effects which carried into the afternoon of the following day. It also appeared to induce mild depressive effects. I was a busy person and while Cetirizine appeared to be effective in controlling the angioedema, it reduced my quality of life too much.

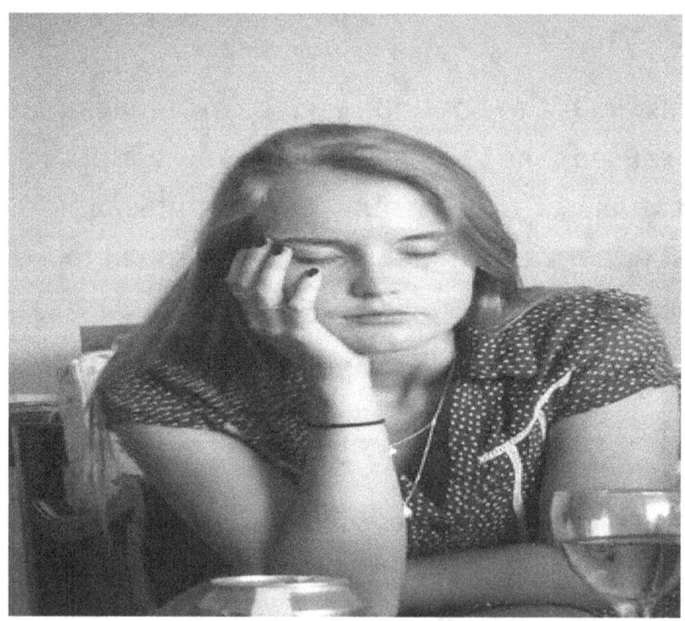

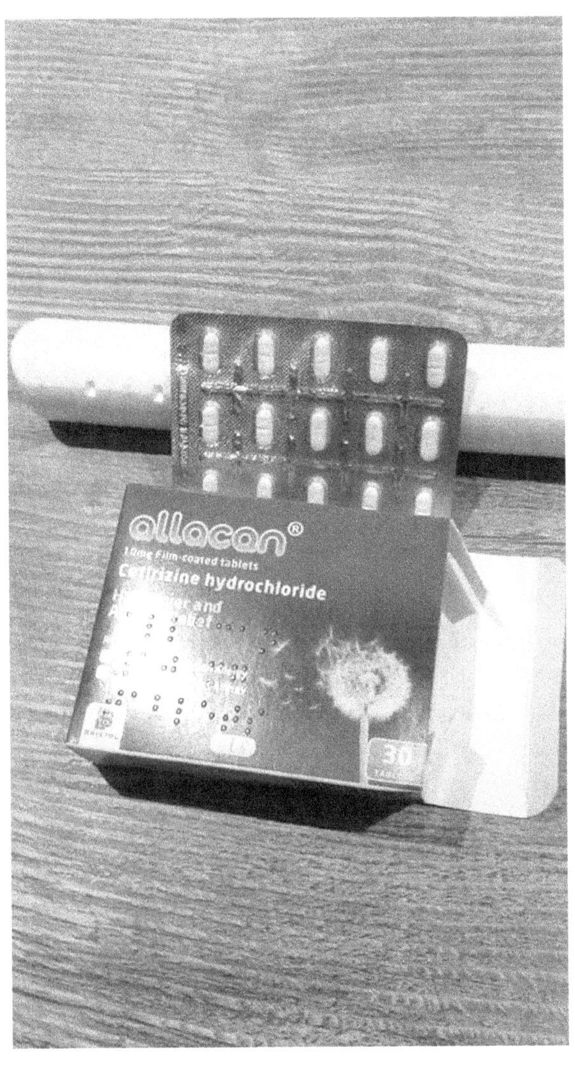

Older generation antihistamines make you sleepy

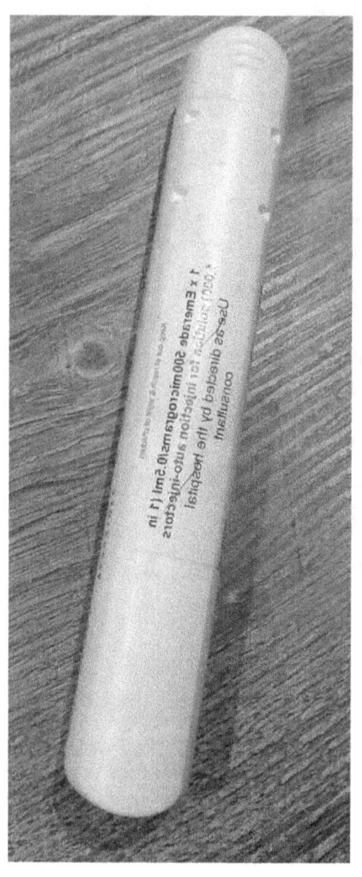

Shortly after my consultation at the immunology clinic I found that my neck was very swollen and I was losing my voice. It didn't really register what it was at the time. I had been given permission to increase my dose of antihistamines but this did not seem make any difference.

I took pictures of the swelling and was given an Epipen next time I went to see the consultant. However, it was impressed that the first line of treatment for angioedema must be antihistamines.

I recall being quite irritated with the way that my condition was being handled. 'Idiopathic' means that a cause – or causes – for a condition hasn't, or haven't, been established; surely further investigation was required.

Prescription medicine in this case does not treat the underlying aetiology merely masks the symptoms. This is, in my view, unsatisfactory. Any medication has potential and unwanted side effects. In addition, any associated conditions still exist – in my case migraine.

Other effects of taking antihistamines long term and these include:

- Dizziness
- Irritability, nervousness
- Changes in vision
- Upset stomach
- Dry mouth, nose, throat
- Constipation
- Sleepiness
- Thicker mucous
- Risk factor for dementia which increases the longer the medication is taken.

The problem with antihistamines is that they can cause also enormous weight gain. This may occur because histamine is an appetite suppressant and once its effect is reduced through the use of antihistamines then, of course, the appetite suppressant effect is lost.

The rapidity with which tissues can swell is amazing. These two pictures were taken of the same person just minutes apart. This is called anaphylaxis which we will look at shortly.

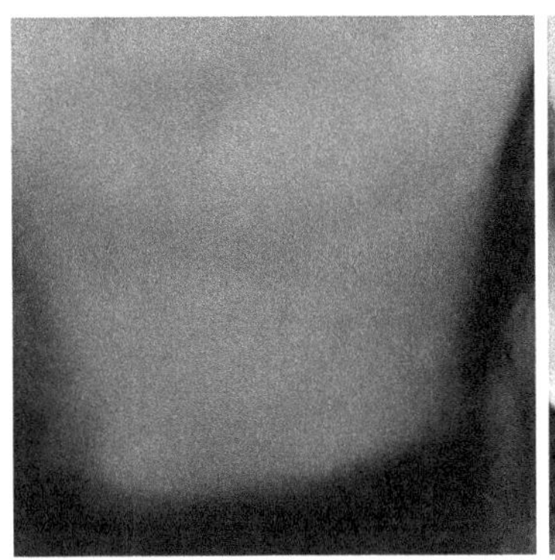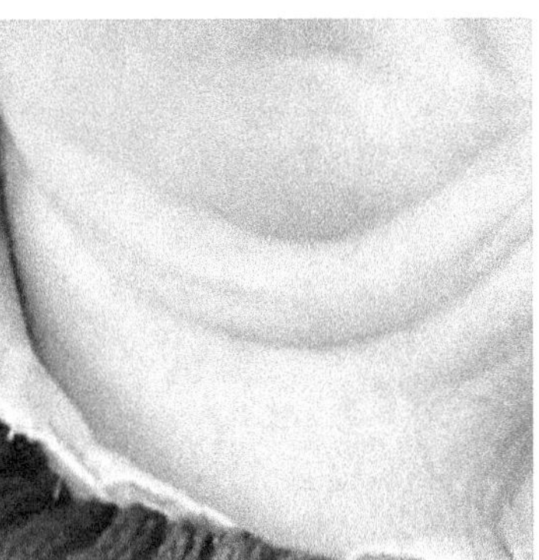

The urticaria which often accompanies angioedema is swelling on the upper layer of the skin. It itches a great deal and sometimes welts appear. Angioedema does not always itch but some people do have itchy angioedema which they find very uncomfortable.

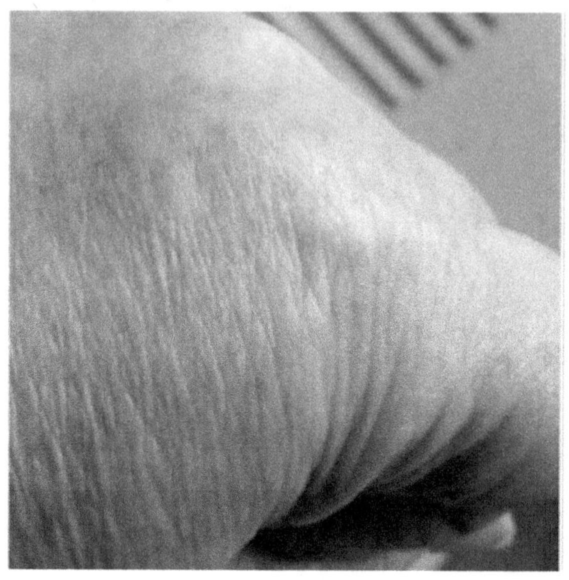

It is not generally long lived but people who are prone to urticaria can suffer from huge areas of red, itchy, swollen skin. Fortunately, antihistamines appear to deal with this quite effectively although it can look quite alarming at the time.

Anaphylaxis

This is a severe allergic reaction and can be potentially fatal if it leads into anaphylactic shock.

The body can react to any number of allergens although common ones are:

- Shellfish
- Bee stings
- Latex
- antibiotics

In severe allergic reactions the blood pressure can plummet suddenly. It can cause breathing problems, shock as well as death.

The epinephrine helps stop the progression of anaphylaxis.

My brother was given aspirin after a routine operation. He went into anaphylactic shock with rapid swelling of tissues. This was the first time this happened. It was fortunate he was in hospital at the time and treatment could be administered immediately.

In spite of yet another familial example, the hospital still denied any familial association.

Clearly, in my brother's case there was a response to a salicylate. Salicylates can trigger a non-allergic mediated response as well as an allergic response through histamine release. The allergic response is more likely to be found in those with asthma. My brother does not have asthma. Salicylates are found in a number of fruit and vegetables. It is fairly impossible to avoid them unless you are very disciplined. However, they include:

- raisins
- prunes
- apricots
- blackberries
- blueberries

- cranberries
- grapes,
- oranges
- strawberries
- pineapple and
- cherries

These are basically foods that I avoided when I was a child purely because they made me feel ill although I could not have explained why.

I still avoid them because they still have the same effect – they make me feel ill. When I tell people that I don't eat fruit (apart from apple and banana) I normally get a finger wagging and a warning that fruit is good for me. Well, not in my case, it isn't!

Histamine Receptors

Histamine receptors are found in many organs in the body such as the lungs, heart, gastrointestinal tract and central nervous system. Histamine receptors are tiny shapes on the cells. They grab onto histamine which directs certain actions in the body. For example, histamine in the gastro intestinal aids the release of stomach acid.

Antihistamines work by blocking these receptors but, in doing so, the blocked receptors cannot grab onto histamine so that specific tissue's function cannot be carried out. However, you do need some histamine to carry out vital functions.

Antihistamines by blocking histamine also block acid release in the stomach and thus are able to address indigestion. However, gut motility is slower and constipation and bloating is a side effect.

In the lungs histamine increases vascular permeability which means that tissues swell up The slightly stuffy feeling you get with hay fever is also due to the same process. The presence of dermatographia (skin writing) also evidences that vascular permeability is occurring. Blocking these receptors can 'dry up' the tissues but mucous membranes are meant to be moist in order to provide a protective barrier. Nevertheless, reducing vascular permeability reduces swelling in tissues. Not only will you feel the difference, your legs will feel lighter, your nose will not be bunged up, you will lose weight and skin writing will disappear in a short term.

Examples of dermographia below. You will see it is quite pronounced.

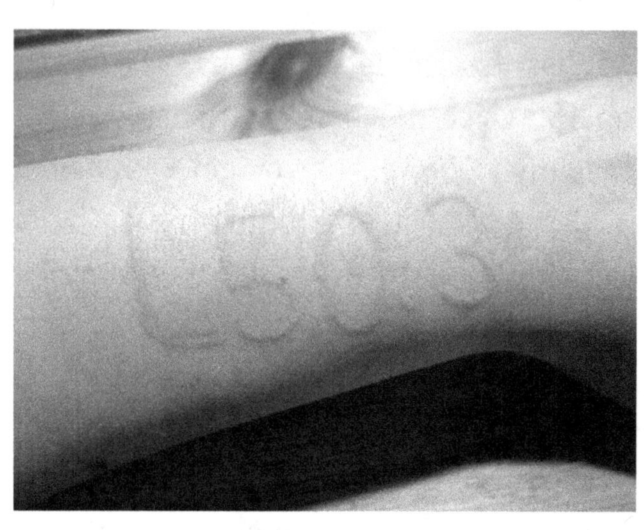

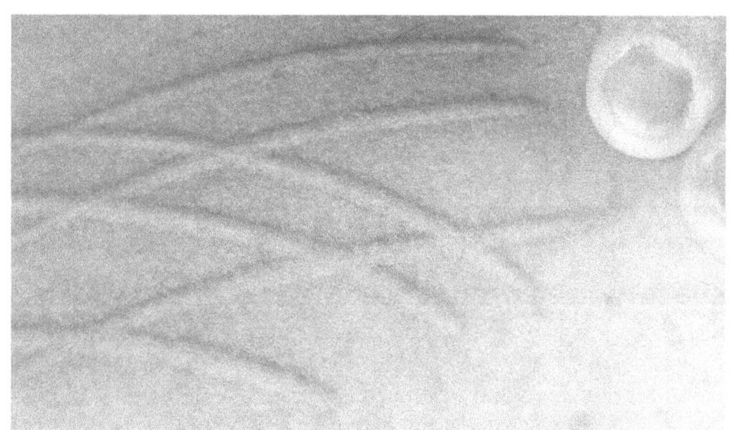

Investigating histamine, looking at where it is made and how it is regulated naturally would give us clues as to how we could treat pathological conditions. Clearly, blocking receptors has unwanted side effects.

Histamine; know thy enemy

Although histamine is associated with negative effects like anaphylaxis an urticaria, it does have a number of important roles to play when it is kept within normal limits. These include:

Regulation of the sleep wake cycle

Enhances cognitive function

Acts a signalling molecule by sending messages between immune system cells to coordinate a defence against invading infection.

It helps regulate body temperature

It helps regulate food intake

It aids memory learning

The impact of too much histamine is – that is when the H1 receptor is activated is:

Low blood pressure

Tachycardia

Vascular permeability

Flushing

Bronchoconstriction

Vasodilation

Itching and weals

H2 receptors

These are found mainly in the stomach and their prime function is to aid the release of acid in order to promote digestion. However, they also help the release of mucus in glands in the airways.

In addition to many of the functions of activated HR1, HR2 can cause headaches.

HR3 receptors are found in the neurons of the central nervous system. As well as regulating histamine they are also involved in the regulation of dopamine, acetylcholine and norepinephrine.

HR4 cells are found in bone marrow and help form some blood cells.

Histamine is found in various parts of the body; as granules in mast cells and basophils but is synthesised from an enzyme L-histidine carboxylase in the neurons of the central nervous system and gastric mucosa.

It is the mast cells that I shall be taking a more in depth look at today. When they detect something harmful, they drop histamine onto it. Bear in mind that there will be numerous mast cells rushing to the scene of injury or harmful invader; it is not a minor action.

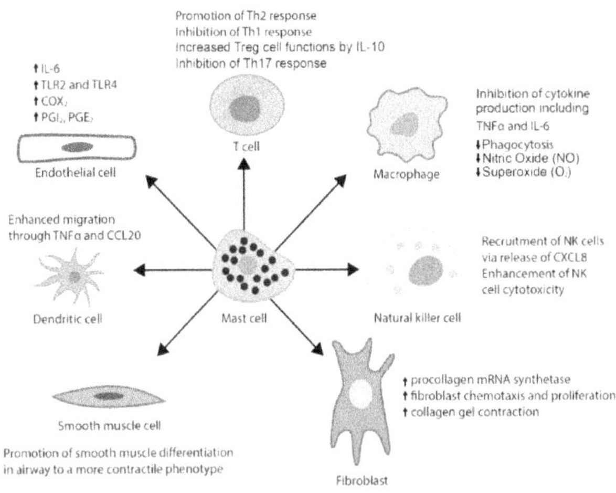

Mast cells have numerous functions including storage and release of histamine granules

it explains why urticaria appears in small patches and very rarely results in an all body urticarial outbreak. Something has been detected in a specific place so mast cells rush to deal with it. Thankfully, histamine has a very short half-life so an isolated invader will result in acute symptoms which will disappear rapidly.

The problem is when there is something in the environment that a sufferer is perpetually in contact with or where the normal brakes regulating histamine fail.

If we can correct the latter then it normally addresses the former, anyway.

Regulation of Histamine levels

The regulation of histamine levels is achieved effectively through the use of nutritional medicine; that is, therapeutic treatment that is within everyone's grasp.

In some unfortunate people the mast cells appear to be very 'twitchy' and tip their contents out at the least little excuse to do so. These mast cells need stabilising or histamine levels need reducing but in a more controlled way without producing the side effects that are associated with antihistamines.

Vitamin C is a natural antihistamine as it helps stabilise mast cells.

Currently, vitamin C ranks 4th on the scale of nutrient deficiencies. This may seem unlikely given that we are encouraged to eat 5 a day and, at one time, 10 a day which should address the needs of most people, you would think. Gene editing more vitamin C into fresh fruit and vegetables was on the cards at one time although given the increase in scurvy one wonders if it was gene edited out.

We are informed that an orange – to take an example – contains about 30mg vitamin C. Perhaps picked off the bush fresh, eaten straightaway and not cooked or stored in anyway would produce this amount but the reality is:

The fruit travels half way around the world

It sits in the supermarket for a long time

It is taken home and sits in a fruit bowl

Vegetables are generally cooked

All of these sound the death knell for vitamin C. By the time you have bought your orange and eaten it, there is probably no vitamin C of any worth left in it.

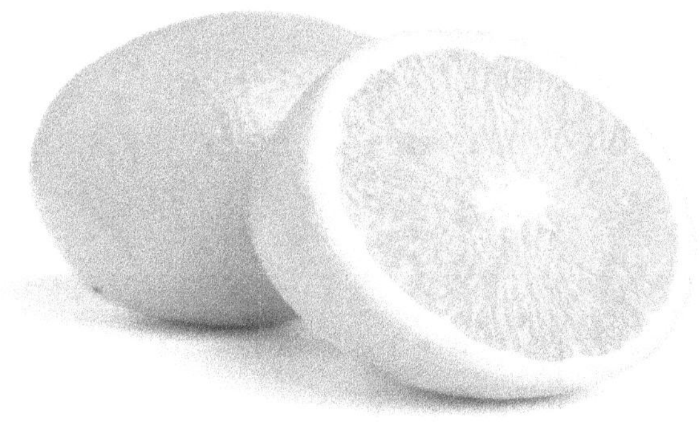

An orange is said to contain 30mg of vitamin C

The current recommendations for vitamin C daily intake are woefully low.

75mg for adult females

90mg for adult males

Just enough to prevent scurvy but not to keep the body ticking over at optimum capacity or stop mast cells from getting twitchy.

Vitamin C is easily destroyed by sunlight and heat.

2g (2000mg) of vitamin C is recommended to address allergies and angioedema but this can be varied to suit the individual. There are a number of flavoured vitamin C tablets which can be dropped into water to make a glass of fizzy fruit drink. They contain 1000mg of vitamin C. As vitamin C is water soluble, any excess is passed out of the body in urine.

The need for vitamin C varies from day to day as it is involved in so many functions. Take, for example, the hugely increased intake needed if you are coming down with a common cold.

Vitamin C is needed to activate immune system cells known as neutrophils; these are one of the first immune system cells that become active when infection first strikes. However, at least 3g (3000mg) of vitamin C is required to activate neutrophils and this does not include the vitamin C that you would need for all the other functions in the body such as helping to stabilise mast cells. Now you can begin to see how inadequate 75mg of vitamin C is as a recommended dietary intake.

Using bowel tolerance is a fairly rough guide although what counts as the amount needed to saturate tissues on one particular day is not necessarily the amount needed for the following day. Stress is known to use vitamin C up rapidly.

Bowel tolerance

Take 2g (2000mg) of vitamin C

If this does not produce a sudden and watery bowel movement, the tissues are not yet saturated.

Continue taking 500mg or 1g (1000mg) every hour until bowel tolerance is found.

Once you have found bowel tolerance, deduct 500mg from the total you have used and this will be your guide for the following day.

However, it is only a guide as requirements can vary so much on a daily basis.

Quercetin

Quercetin helps to stabilise histamine levels in a similar way to that of vitamin C. Quercetin is a flavone, a polyphenol which is found in many edible plants such as in cauliflower, broccoli and green tea as well as foods belonging to the allium family such as garlic and onions. These type of flavonoids contain colourful pigments.

I love onions and add them to as many dishes as I can. Thus, even if many fruit and vegetables are depleted in vitamin C, there is still value in them in the form of quercetin for reducing histamine levels.

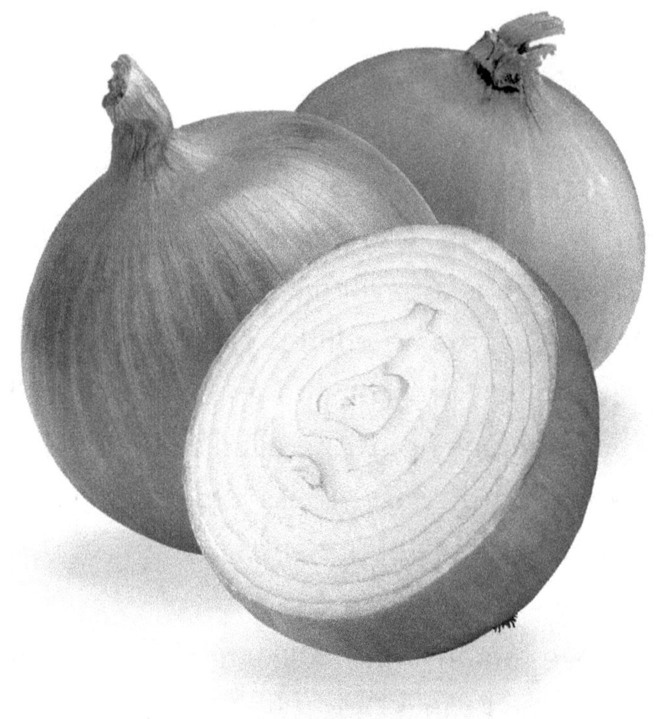

onions contain quercetin which helps to quell histamine levels by stabilising mast cells

Long term use of high dose quercetin is probably not advisable. The amount that you would obtain from a daily intake of fresh fruit and vegetables is useful however most quercetin supplements tend to come in dosages of 500mg. Was this based on any adequate research or did it just look like a nice round amount?

If we look into quercetin further, we find that, like vitamin C it has anti-inflammatory and antioxidant capacity. However, these tests are carried out in the laboratory and what occurs there does not necessarily occur in the body.

Supplements of quercetin are often combined with bromelain which is an enzyme found in pineapple.

Quercetin is associated with common side effects like headache and upset stomach. In very high doses quercetin is known to damage the kidneys.

The recommendation is to take periodic breaks when taking quercetin in supplement form when taken in large doses. Increasing fruit and vegetables is preferable.

It is also recommended that pregnant and breastfeeding women should avoid supplemental quercetin.

Further, quercetin may possibly interact with

Anticoagulants like warfarin and increase the risk of bleeding

Antibiotics and reduce their effectiveness

Corticosteroids by slowing down the breakdown of these so that they stay in the body long

This is not a definitive list.

We have looked at two nutrients which you can supplement which help stabilise mast cells. Does the body manufacture any substance which helps to stabilise histamine? It is to this; I shall now turn.

.

Diamine Oxidase (DAO)

DAO is a vital enzyme which is found in the digestive tract. It is useful for those with histamine intolerance which, as we have seen, can be responsible for migraines and headaches, skin conditions and gut problems.

Some people are unfortunate that they don't produce DAO and will experience histamine intolerance so that a wide range of foods cause problems.

These include:

Nuts

soybeans

milk

shellfish

pineapple

mushrooms

chocolate

oily fish

A histamine intolerance is not the same as an allergy. Allergies are generally linked to one specific food and the immune system, including an immunoglobulin E (IgE) while a histamine intolerance cannot be pinpointed to one food; it occurs when the mast cells aren't stable. Further, the body makes histamine endogenously in the gastrointestinal tract. Excess histamine when released from cells will cause these symptoms

Migraines

Nausea and vomiting

Bloating, stomach pain, constipation and gas

Flu like pain

Stuffy nose

Urticaria

Wheezing

Faint, feeling faint and dizziness

Psoriasis

It may be necessary to supplement with DAO or increase foods that contain DAO.

There are encouraging results in those who took supplemental DAO for gut issues. It appears to heal the gut lining. The general recommended dosage is approximately 4.2 mg three times daily.

It is considered quite expensive although an excellent source of DAO is olive oil.

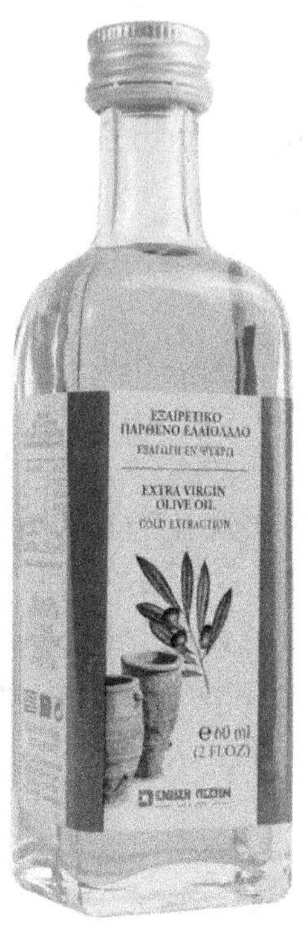

Olive oil contains good amounts of DAO.

As well as the enzyme DAO, an amino acid known as histidine has proven to be useful in treating allergies. It is worth learning a little more about its therapeutic potential.

Histidine.

Histidine (do not confuse this with histamine) has been studied and found to be effective in treating allergies. This study[1] found:

- A role of therapeutic usefulness of the amino acid histidine is indicated in allergic and *related* conditions. (Therefore it has potential for idiopathic angioedema).
- Histidine is antagonistic to histamine and plays an important part in histamine-adrenalin balance in shock.
- Histidine produces a feeling of well-being and energy that could be useful in the care of post-operative patients and the treatment of shock.
- Further study of histidine enrichment of parenterally administered protein hydrolysates as blood substitutes is being conducted.

---

[1] https://link.springer.com/article/10.1007/BF02997423

Histidine can be found in a variety of foods. These include:

- Dairy
- Meat
- Eggs
- Cheese
- Fish
- Mushrooms
- Cauliflower
- Potatoes

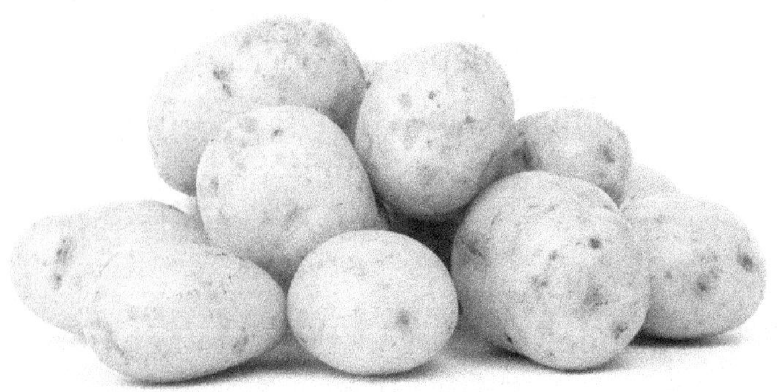

Potatoes contain histidine

Histidine can also be obtained online or in good health food stores. It comes in powder or tablet form mainly. It tends to be one of the more expensive amino acids but, it won't work out any more expensive than any over the counter medication you buy for any allergy related condition.

Histidine powder can also be added to neutral pH ointment and applied to areas which are itchy as it has calming properties.

Be guided by the dosage on the packet if you use the powdered or tablet form

I have certainly found histidine useful and have not needed to use my Epipen since introducing more histidine containing foods as a prophylactic treatment for my condition.

There are other amino acids which have therapeutic potential, in treating allergies; one such amino acid is glycine.

Glycine

Glycine, the smallest amino acid, has been found in studies[2] to ameliorate the effects of cow's milk and the acute allergic responses it can produce in some susceptible people. The findings supported the hypothesis that the oral intake of glycine could prevent a cow's milk allergy.

Glycine can be obtained in granule form. It looks like sugar and is sweet like sugar and so will be readily accepted by babies.

The RDI of glycine is 1.5-3g daily but it is preferable if the glycine is obtained from food one of which the best sources is bone broth. Any slow cooked meat, like brisket, which forms a gelatinous mass in the gravy when cooled also contains glycine.

Wine gums used to be excellent for soothing stomachs due to their high gelatine content (gelatine contains a high percentage of glycine)

---

[2]

https://www.sciencedirect.com/science/article/pii/S0271531718300095

but some wine gums now contain ingredients which aren't gelatine.

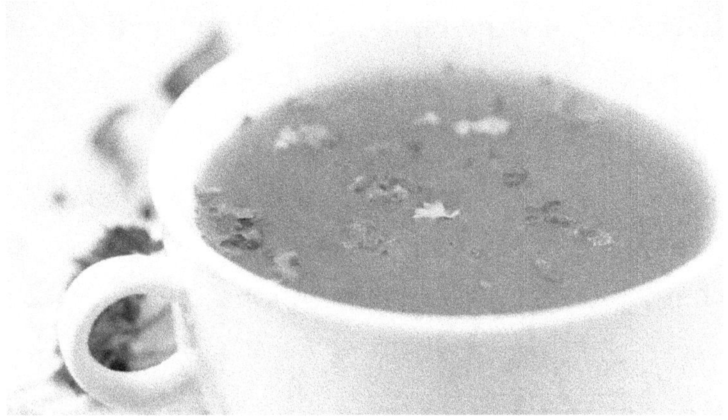

Bone broth contains good amounts of glycine

Nettles also have anti-inflammatory properties. People often drink nettle tea if they have allergies. It is quite easy to make your own by drying the leaves before using them exactly as you would ordinary tea.

Nettle and potato soup used to be popular in the immediate and post war years. It is a shame that this nutritious food has gone out of fashion since its benefits extend far beyond its effects on allergies.

The amino acid, taurine

Taurine is a conditional amino acid which means that generally the body makes it but, at times of injury or illness or ageing, then we require more than the body can supply.

The daily requirement for taurine is 3g but an average diet consumes only 59mg - far below that which is required for optimum health.

The countries that have the diets with the highest amounts of taurine also have greater longevity than those with lesser amounts in their diet.

Taurine helps to keep the fluid inside and outside the cell in balance. People have remarked that they have found that after two days of taurine supplementation of 3g daily (in divided doses) that the majority of oedema had disappeared.

As it has other beneficial effects and long term studies do not find any contra-indications for taking taurine long term, then It will be on my list of supplements especially as it appeared to deal effectively with the swelling of angioedema.

Taurine is made from sulphur containing amino acids. This could be a problem for people who are intolerant to sulphur but, if not, then it is one amino acid that I feel should be given more importance than it has.

Taurine is found in fish products.

It's role in treating allergic reactions reaches beyond its anti-inflammatory and antioxidant properties. There is research that shows that it can prevent the infiltration of mast cells into the nasal cavity. Further, it reduces another immune cell, known as eosinophils from similar.

Eosinophils are little known work horses of the immune system. Kept in check they keep you healthy. Their functions include;

Fight infection

Help repair tissue

 Modulate inflammation

Required in the formation of organs. For example, they help in the development of mammary glands required during and after pregnancy.

They trap foreign particles and kill cells

They are antiparasitic and have bactericidal activity

They are involved in the immediate allergic reaction helping to degrade and inactivate substances like histamine released by mast cells.

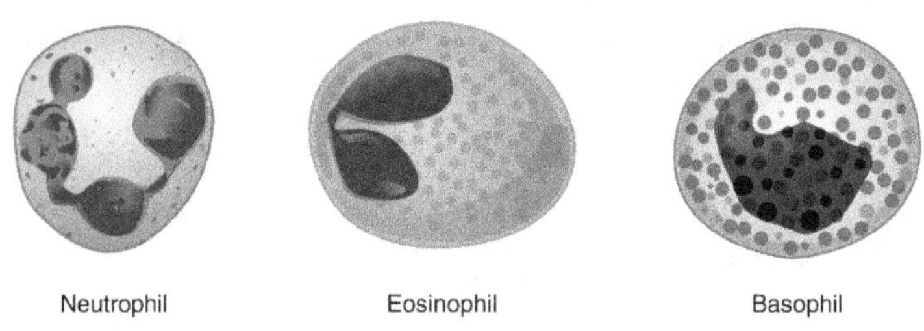

Various immune system cells involved in intolerance and allergic reactions

Basophils, which have already been mentioned tend to be involved in later stages of the allergic response.

Eosinophils live in the gastrointestinal tract but will migrate to sites which are inflamed due to allergy.

The immune system can become very enthusiastic when it detects a foreign body and taurine can help modulate an over-enthusiastic reaction.

The role of vitamin D

A number of important studies have highlighted the important role that vitamin D has to play in reducing angioedema, urticaria and other allergic types responses. The study is important because recurrent episodes of flushing, urticaria and angioedema are symptomatic of many conditions. These include cardiovascular, gastrointestinal, endocrine, neurological, dermatological and allergic causes although this is not a definitive list.

The study described below involves a novel therapeutic approach. Such is its significance for the conditions I have just mentioned, that I have described it in some detail below.

Vitamin D and Mast Cell Activation Syndrome

The study[3] involved a 60 year old woman who had recurrent episodes of flushing, urticaria and angioedema. She had presented to the allergy clinic after visiting the emergency department for 'total body flushing' about an hour after eating wheat crackers, cheese and decaffeinated tea.

This wasn't the first time that she had presented to the emergency department with generalised flushing. There had been some abdominal discomfort.

Her medical history included:

- asthma
- fibromyalgia
- osteoarthritis
- migraines
- hyperlipidaemia
- hypothyroidism

Her medications included: sumatripan (for migraines), fexofenadine, (antihistamine),

---

[3] https://www.ncbi.nlm.nih.gov/pmc/articles/PMC4405605/

albuterol (for asthma), levothyroxine (for thyroid) and fluoxetine (an antidepressant).

She had had syncopal episodes. Syncope is a temporary loss of consciousness that is related to insufficient blood supply to the brain. It is also referred to as fainting.

Her examination was unremarkable. At the time she presented to the clinic she did not show any of the symptoms which were in evidence when she attended the emergency department.

The patient was given cetirizine 10mg nightly as well as an Epipen. Naturally, she was told to avoid anything which might disagree with her. Nevertheless, she continued to have approximately three episodes annually. These generally occurred when she was preparing her normal meals.

In spite of being prescribed further medication including ranitidine and Montelukast, none of these additional interventions appeared to change the course of the disease.

Finally, some out-patient work up also revealed severe vitamin D deficiency. Her levels were 6ng/mL where the reference range is 25-100 ng/ml.

She was treated with 50,000 IU weekly with a repeat of this until at twelve weeks, her levels were 47ng/ml. At this point she received 50,000 IU's on alternate weeks.

Over the following year, she did not have any episodes of flushing, angioedema or anaphylactic reactions. There have been some minor urticarial type lesions but they were intermittent and self-limiting.

It is not surprising that vitamin D is able to control Mast Cell Activation Syndrome, as described above, for it is an important immune system regulator.

Mast cell syndrome (MCS) means that mast cells release inflammatory mediators in larger amounts and more often than required. Mast cells release a substance known as histamine which makes blood vessels leaky. This leakiness allows cells to pass through the blood vessels to the site of injury. However, the leakiness causes swelling, redness and itchiness along the way.

How vitamin D_3 – the active form of vitamin D – stabilises mast cells, appears to take more than one route. Vitamin D appears to regulate a substance known as COX which is an enzyme which produces prostaglandins. Therefore, vitamin D can sabotage the production of prostaglandin.

When vitamin D was taken for six weeks, it was found[4] to cause programmed cell death in a cell model. It also inhibited the differentiation and maturation of mast cell precursors.

Mast cells are found in bone marrow as mast cell precursors. They mature at peripheral sites provided a substance known as Stem Cell Factor is available.

---

[4] Conti P, Kempuraj D. Impact of vitamin D on mast cell activity, immunity and inflammation. Journal of Food and Nutrition Research 2016: 4(1), 33-39.

Although we hear a lot about inflammatory mediators there are also **anti-**inflammatory mediators. Two of these, known as interleukin–4 and interleukin-10, which help to regulate inflammation are produced in greater quantities by the action of vitamin D in the body.

It is clear that vitamin D acts on many levels to regulate mast cells and make sure that the distressing effects of mast cell activation syndrome do not occur.

There are many, many mast cell triggers and these include:

- heat, cold, sudden temperature changes
- stress from various sources
- exercise
- odours
- NSAID's, antibiotics, dyes among others
- fatigue
- insect venom
- sun/sunlight
- infections

The above is not an exhaustive list.

The sun can   destabilise mast cells in some susceptible people who have a cholinergic angioedema   but the vitamin D it helps synthesise can regulate mast cells in most people. Genes make the difference.

The problem with making sure that we have sufficient vitamin D is that it is not found in many food types. Oily fish is a good source and vitamin D is added to some, but not all, cereals.

Eggs also contain some vitamin D but you would need to eat 80 daily to get your recommended daily allowance of vitamin D. This would provide the very minimum of vitamin D that was required daily.

Our main source of vitamin D is the sun. During the 1950's there was an epidemic of rickets due to lack of vitamin D in the diet. At that time, it was not added to cereals and very few children liked oily fish.

There is one source of plant based vitamin D and that is irradiated mushrooms; that is mushrooms left in sunlight to absorb their rays.

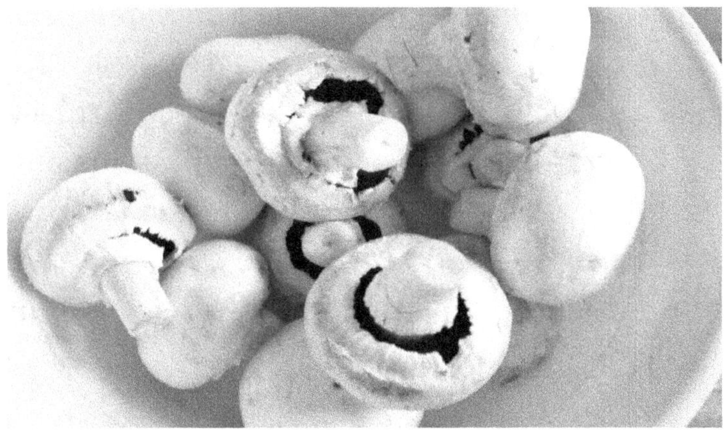

Irradiated mushrooms will contain vitamin D

Children were dosed daily with cod liver oil to stave off rickets. Lining up for a teaspoonful of it daily, was part of the ritual of family life in the 1950's.

Rickets – since daily dosing of cod liver was abandoned - has returned once more, allergies are rife in all its forms, yet when I was a child, I did not know of anyone who had any allergic type condition.

 Children's diets have not improved; children tend to spend a lot more time indoors out of the sunlight and its healing rays. If they do venture out, they are immediately covered in high factor sun cream and wide brimmed hats. Their ability to make their own vitamin D – which is what nature intended - has virtually sunk to zero. Meanwhile, eczema, asthma and hay fever- as well as angioedema-is on the rise. It is not surprising when our bodies do not have the nutrients needed for the essential task of regulating mast cells.

MAST CELL

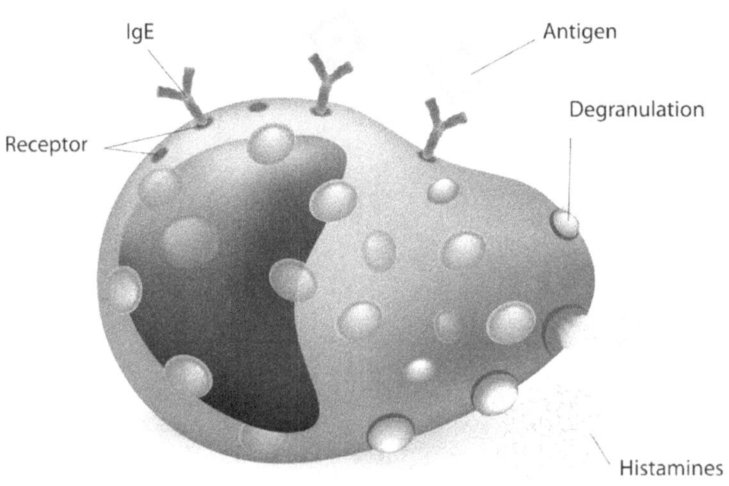

5

Although I am an outdoor person, it is harder to synthesise vitamin D from the sun as you age; it is also harder to absorb vitamin D from the diet.

I used to take 4000 IU's of vitamin D from October until the following May at which point the sun's rays became more potent

Vitamin D continues to be a poorly understood vitamin in many respects given the impact it has on your overall health. Its strength lies in its

---

5 https://healthimpactnews.com/2018/are-vaccines-linked-to-increase-in-mast-cell-disease-and-allergies/

ability as an immune system regulator so at times of

- injury
- infection
- illness

then the beneficial impact that vitamin D could have on these conditions should not be overlooked.

Vitamin D can be applied topically to itchy or reddened areas associated with any of the above mentioned conditions. Some soft gels can be opened and the contents rubbed onto the skin for rapid relief. Try a small patch area first; it is still possible to react to the soft gel capsule some of which will be mixed in with its contents. However, in the main, it should be ingested in diet, supplement form and by the action of sunlight on the skin so that its far reaching effects can impact on every part of the body, within the body, which is its normal mode of operating.

Special attention must be made by those with darker skins as their absorption of vitamin D is reduced. Further, the elderly, housebound or those with gastrointestinal problems are also likely to be vitamin D deficient.

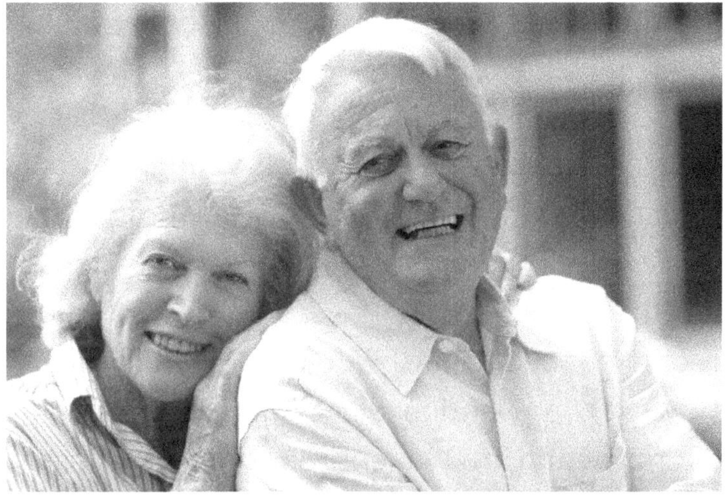

Elderly do not synthesise vitamin D from the sun's rays efficiently, neither do they absorb it as well as they would have done when younger.

It is estimated that 80% of all people worldwide will be deficient in this vitamin. While not all of these people will be symptomatic of non-hereditary angioedema or allergy due to genetic influences, there will be some detriment although this may not reveal itself immediately.

It is better to take responsibility for your health and insist on regular checks for vitamin D status especially if there are signs, however mild, of life-threatening conditions like angioedema.

Most supplemental forms of vitamin D only provide 400 international units (iu's) of vitamin D. This recommended daily intake was adopted in the 1950's. It was the lowest dose recommended that would prevent rickets. However, prevention of rickets and promoting overall health are two entirely different things.

There needs to be a rethink on the recommended daily allowance for vitamin D especially when individuals have mast cell activation disorders or similar. It is such a simple potential treatment that it has been overlooked as many too 'obvious' potential treatments generally are.

Angioedema 'burns itself out.' It is reported in some respected journals. I do not think that there has been much consideration about what does cause angioedema to burn itself out. Clearly, something does. There are reasons why events occur regardless whether we are aware of or understand them. We need to develop a little more curiosity and a more open mind. Too readily we dismiss what research hasn't already opened doors to rather than exploring a line of interest ourselves.

It is not without the realm of possibility that:

Someone has unwittingly changed their diet and decreased intake of histamine containing foods or

Has been on a foreign holiday which has topped up their vitamin D levels

or increased DAO in their diet by adopting the Mediterranean diet in an effort to eat more healthily

Of course, prescribing vitamin D does not make huge profits for pharmaceutical companies. The link between vitamin D deficiency and allergy does not appear to have reached the GP surgery. Always……. always such a limited range of tests and when they come back negative, a completely inappropriate treatment will be prescribed because patients expect to be prescribed something.

The signs of vitamin D deficiency include:

 Deep bone pain

Muscle weakness and spasms

Tremors

Waddling gait

Fatigue

Depression

Hair loss

Repeated infections

Appetite loss

I have no doubt that there are many treatments out there for currently 'untreatable' conditions but they never move from concept to the clinic because of their unprofitability.

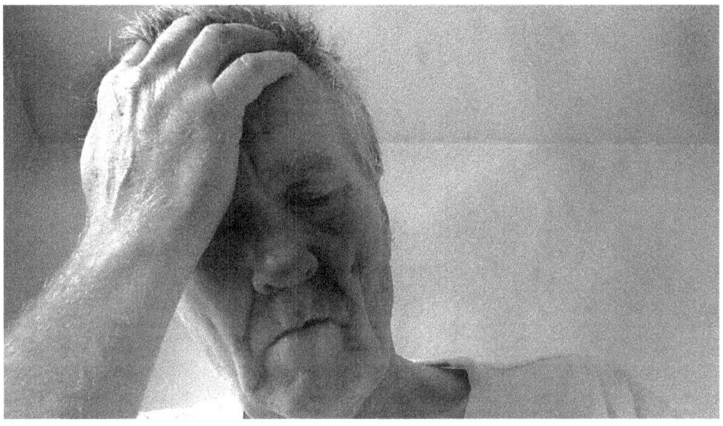

Fatigue is a sign of vitamin D deficiency

.

Returning to the subject of nitrates

A number of foods that make people feel ill and rapidly bring on a migraine contain nitrates. These include:

 dark chocolate

red wine

citrus fruits

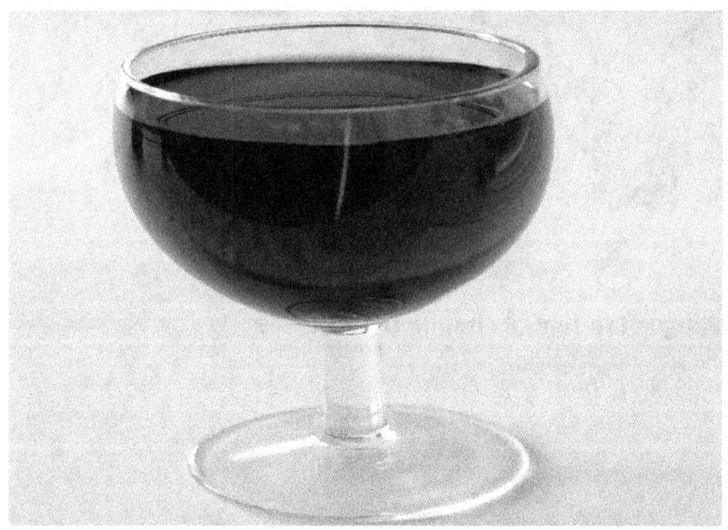

Red wine contains nitrates

Although red wine and citrus fruits contain salicylates they also contain nitrates. dark chocolate does not contain salicylates. Salicylates are not associated with migraine, nitrates are.

Chocolate and cocoa do not normally bring on urticaria but ingesting them rapidly brings on migraine in susceptible people as does the nitrate-containing citrus fruit and red wine.

Most people will avoid these foods without realising why. It is not that people don't like them as such, but they make them feel ill and they come to associate certain foods with this.

Nitrates are in a diverse range of foods. Small amounts do not appear to cause too many problems but go beyond a specific amount — which differs in everyone susceptible to them. and the headaches, facial and oesophageal swelling will occur. For example, I can probably eat half a small square of dark chocolate and not have a migraine. However, more than that and I will get some unpleasant swelling in my throat, some facial swelling and a feeling of being stuffed up.

A couple of hours beyond that I will get the familiar feeling of an impending migraine and the accompanying   inability to cope with light or noise. For me there isn't a feel good factor in eating foods high in nitrates.

The antidote to the effects of nitrates is to avoid foods that contain large amounts of these. For me this included removing:

- Red wine
- Citrus foods
- Dark chocolate
- Processed meat such as
- Bacon
- Ham
- Salami
- Corned beef
- Hot dogs
- Pate
- Canned meats

- Smoked salmon

- Jerky

- Dried fish

This may initially look like a huge list and you may wonder what there is left that you can eat but any fresh meat – chicken, beef, pork and lamb – the mainstay of the great British Sunday roast is fine.

Avoid smoked foods – they are high in nitrates – red wine, beers, chocolate. Many tinned products will list nitrates as an additive so it is worth looking at the ingredients list on the label.

 There are also plenty of lists of high nitrate foods available online. My guess is that most people who find that nitrates produce unwanted effects are already avoiding foods that produce those symptoms but lists are useful if you are keeping a food diary and are wanting to find associations between foods that appear to bring on angioedema.

This may be harder than is first realised. It is easy to identify facial swelling or other external swelling but not so easy to identify swelling of the lining of the gastrointestinal tract.

Those symptoms that have been experienced may have already been given a label such as irritable bowel syndrome. However, a syndrome is just a collection of symptoms. It does not tell us what the cause is nor indeed how we can treat it. When we have a label for a collection of symptoms it has a tendency to become part of our identity – something that we are reluctant to let go of so that we can re-examine it. However, it is always better to do so. Symptoms do not just occur without a cause. There is a reason why they appear and the exploration of why they occur should be a joint effort between patient and medic.

In our hunt for nutritionally therapeutic responses to

Zinc

Zinc is an essential trace mineral which has approximately 400 different functions in the body which include:

Wound healing

Blood clotting

The smooth running of the thyroid

The smooth running of the immune system

The sensation of smell and taste

The synthesis of macromolecules like proteins

Responding to histamine intolerance

We have already learned that DAO is essential for breaking down excessive histamine but it is also true that any enzyme or nutrient does not work in isolation from others. The body is a hive of activity provided it has been given all that it needs to run smoothly and is not infiltrated by too many toxins.

Zinc works alongside DAO helping to break down histamine.

In the stomach, zinc is better at reducing stomach acid than the over the counter and prescription PPI's and other antacids.

Zinc helps to increase the gastric mucosal barrier by increasing the amount produced.

Moreover, zinc helps to lower acid output in gastric secretion.

Zinc deficiency is rife nowadays; plant based diets contain little usable zinc since the phytates in plants grab hold onto zinc and prevent its absorption.

Although zinc deficiencies can produce many apparently unrelated symptoms, due to genetic diversity, not everyone will show all the symptoms and some may show more than others.

Symptoms of zinc deficiency include:

Skin changes which look like eczema but will not respond to steroids or moisturisers. Skin will look cracked and take on a shiny smooth 'glazed appearance.' This normally affects the mouth, hands and nappy area.

Hair loss

Loss of smell and taste

Frequent infections

Wounds which take ages to heal

 Diarrhoea

Normal growth and development is compromised which may mean people reach puberty later than that which is accepted

The best sources of zinc are to be found in animal proteins.

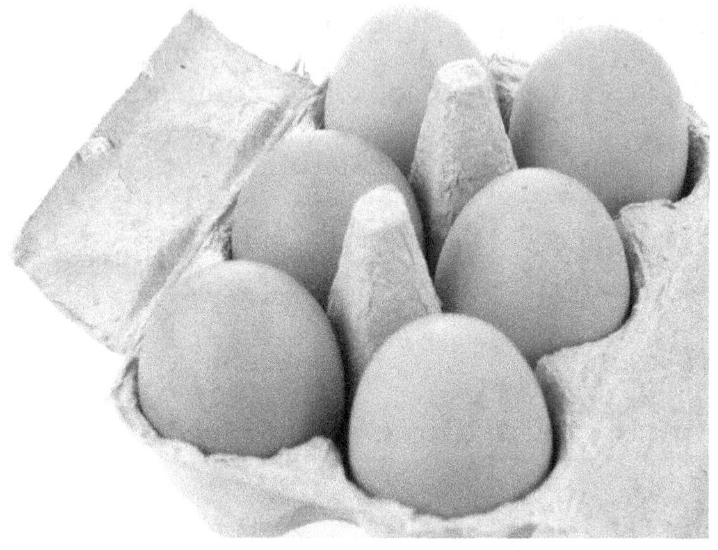

Eggs are a good source of protein

Other nutrients in which a deficiency may be a risk factor for histamine intolerance

It cannot be repeated enough that nutrients do not work in isolation. If we talk about the DAO enzyme and do not have sufficient knowledge to understand that vitamin C and copper are vital for this enzyme, then we will not seek to address any deficiency and therefore histamine will not break down enough and symptoms of intolerance will occur in susceptible people.

Vitamin B6 is vital to aid DAO to degrade histamine but, in order to be activated, vitamin B6 needs a sufficient supply of vitamin B2 (riboflavin).

Riboflavin is found in good amounts in milk but milk drinking has fallen out of popularity and we find the supermarkets stocking some form of plant based milk trying to convince us that it is better for us. Rarely do people ever take time out to actually look at this to ascertain it is true.

Sometimes the benefits are touted as 'lowering cholesterol' where the vast majority of people have bought the lie that cholesterol is some form of demonic substance that may wend its way into the arteries and clog them up. Rarely it is mentioned that cholesterol is healing, that most of your brain is made up of it, that those with higher levels live longer and are less likely to die from respiratory or gastrointestinal infection. The list goes on but from the time we were born it was inculcated in us that cholesterol is bad.

Magnesium is another of those nutrients that we tend to be deficient in. Like many other nutrients it is associated with allergies because too little magnesium means that histamine metabolism and immune function work below optimum levels.

Here is yet another mineral required in the synthesis of the enzyme DAO, which when in short supply enables histamine levels to rise.

It's ability to reduce spasm and open airways is particularly useful in cases of bronchoconstriction.

Magnesium ointment is also helpful in cases of skin complaints where there is an allergen or some non IgE substance involved.

Good sources of magnesium are to be found in:

Green leafy vegetables

Whole grains

Nuts

Fish

Dairy

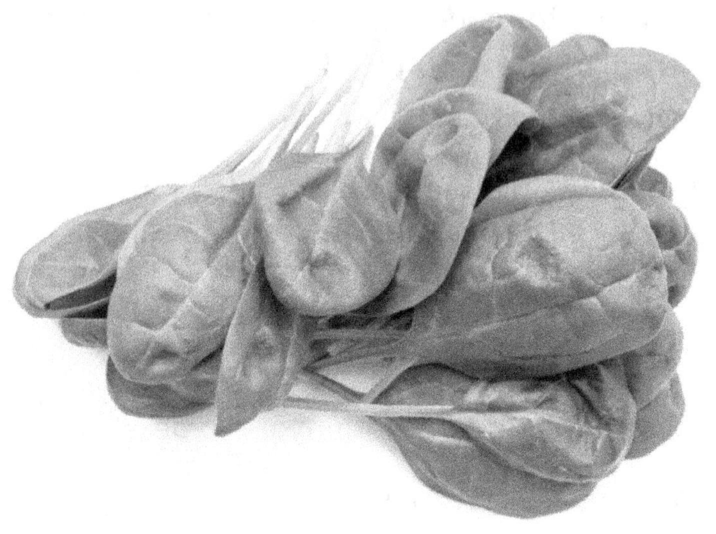

Spinach contains good amounts of magnesium.

It is easily flushed out of the body during diuretic use or in the peculiar habit of drinking two litres of water a day, regardless of whether your body needs it or not.

Antacids will reduce its absorption.

Signs and symptoms of a magnesium deficiency include:

Loss of appetite

Muscle spasms

Arrhythmia

Nausea and vomiting

Tics

Fatigue

Weakness

Numbness and tingling

Seizures

Personality changes

Nystagmus (abnormal eye movements)

Those who are particularly susceptible to magnesium deficiency are those with coeliac disease, alcoholism, type 2 diabetes, those who have had gastrointestinal surgery as well as those on certain medications.

If you must take a supplement, then these forms are better absorbed:

Magnesium citrate

Magnesium gluconate

Magnesium lactate

Riboflavin; a non-allergic, non-intolerance reason for throat swelling

Although we have covered allergies and intolerances fairly well, there are nutrient deficiencies which do not fit into either of those categories although their side effects may immediately lead people to think it is one or the other.

When results come back from various tests and there is no clear indication of what is causing the symptoms then it is labelled 'idiopathic' which simply means, 'We have no idea what is causing it.'

This can be frustrating for the patient who thinks the GP thinks they are making it up.

In some cases, the GP may well think this and slots the patient into 'mental health' in which case they will be asked if anything is causing stress in their life.

In reality, I do not know of anyone who does not suffer stress at any point in their lives. It is a hazard of living and when we have had time to think about the stress and deal with it, then something else will rear its head and we will learn, in time, to overcome that. Most everyday stresses do not need medicating.

Nevertheless, on stating you feel stressed (as you remember the parking ticket you got), the GP will offer you anti-depressants.

If nutrient deficiencies are tested for then it will be a very narrow range of such depending on how easy and cost effective, it is to do so.

Iron and vitamin D status are high on the list of easy and cheap ones to test for but riboflavin is not. However, as you read on you will realise that when it comes to oedematous throat swelling, it should be prioritised; certainly so if a diagnosis of an idiopathic angioedema is given.

Riboflavin deficiency

Riboflavin, also known as vitamin B2, is not as well-known as its sister, vitamin B12 or thiamine (B1) which is rapidly gaining credibility for its ability to reverse dementia, nevertheless its importance is not in doubt.

Riboflavin deficiency is said to be rare but it is only as rare as the motivation and ability of people able to detect it.

It is produced by bacteria in the large intestine which produces free riboflavin. This is then absorbed but the amount depends on diet. Far less is produced on a diet that is mainly carnivorous.

A deficiency is also known as ariboflavinosis and although this can occur due to inadequate intake – and this would be the most common cause – thyroid hormone insufficiency is one condition which can also cause a deficiency.

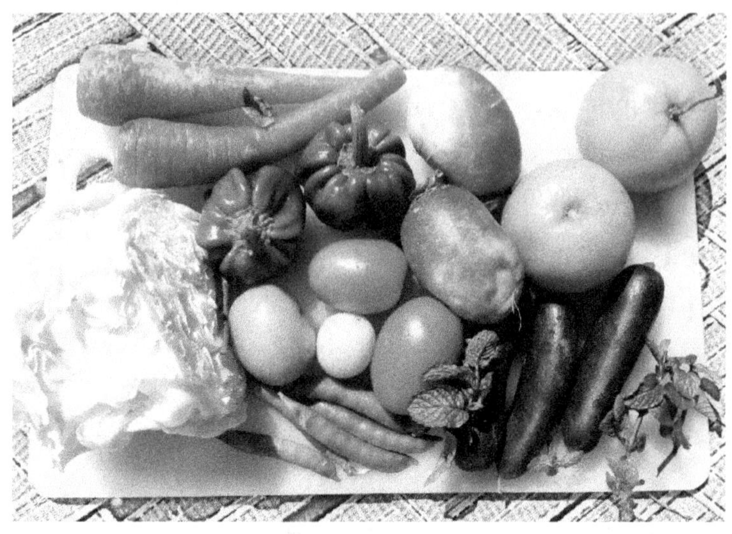

A plant based diet is beneficial to the synthesis of riboflavin

The signs and symptoms of riboflavin deficiency are varied and include:

Hyperaemia – this can also occur without riboflavin deficiency and occurs due to increased blood flow to various parts of the body which may occur when you have been soaking in a warm bath or rubbing hands when they are cold.

Angular stomatitis which are lesions at the corners of the mouth

Cheilosis - swollen cracked lips

Hair loss

Degeneration of the liver

Itchy red eyes

Degeneration of the central nervous system

Anaemia and cataracts (cataracts form after severe and prolonged riboflavin deficiency and rarely is this reversed).

Sore throat

Swollen throat and mouth

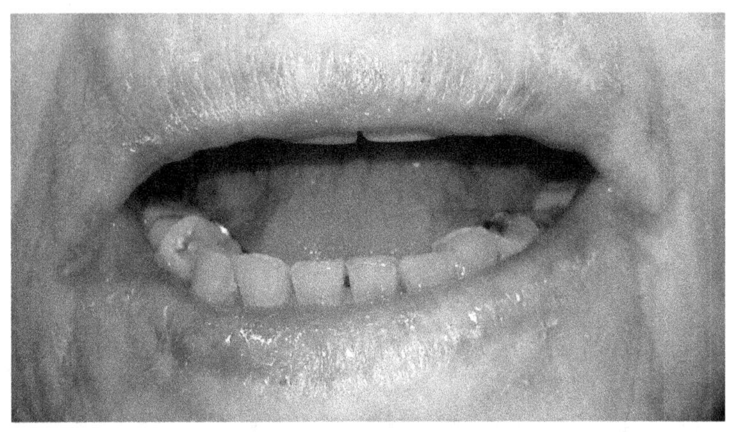

Angular stomatitis   is a symptom of riboflavin deficiency

It is the last mentioned symptoms that we are interested in.

Swollen throat and mouth due to riboflavin deficiency looks very similar to idiopathic angioedema especially when the angular stomatitis may be missing. When you are on the threshold of a riboflavin deficiency, it is possible some days to have a diet which takes you over the amount needed in which case the symptoms will appear to go. However, should you return to a diet which supplies little riboflavin after that, the symptoms will return. It is not unlike the pattern of idiopathic angioedema.

This begs the question is idiopathic angioedema a manifestation of   a nutritional deficiency? After all, not all the symptoms need to be present?

Riboflavin is easily destroyed by sunlight. Housewives would take their milk in immediately it was delivered by the local milkman to preserve the riboflavin and vitamin C content. Otherwise, milk bottle shaped containers which cloaked the milk from the sun were used.

Unfortunately, anticholinergic medications which are used to treat a wide variety of conditions block absorption of riboflavin.

Anti cholinergic medications block a chemical found in the brain called acetylcholine. Acetylcholine is aids muscle movements which are not under our control like peristalsis, the action of the gut as well as other bodily functions.

Anticholinergic drugs are useful in treating

Overactive bladder but too much can delay voiding

Asthma

Motion sickness

Gastrointestinal spasms although too high a dose of anticholinergic drugs can cause constipation.

The point is that where it was rare to find a riboflavin deficiency given the number of anticholinergic drugs there are, it is highly likely that riboflavin deficiency is not as rare as has been mooted.

Even a diet high in riboflavin is not going to work if it cannot be absorbed in the gut.

The recommendations for daily amounts of riboflavin at the moment, for adults, are:

Men 1.3mg daily

Women 1.1mg

Pregnant women 1.3mg

Breast feeding women 1.7mg

However, many of the recommended daily intakes for vitamins have recently been found to be too low. They were set at amounts which were the lowest amount to prevent a deficiency disease but did not reach levels which promoted overall health.

The best sources are dairy products, many of which are sold in opaque containers in order to preserve the vitamin B2.

Other good sources are:

Mushrooms

Brewer's yeast

Nutritional yeast and nutritional yeast flakes

Whole grain and wheat germ

Almonds

Soybeans

Brussels sprouts

Spinach

broccoli

However, all these should be stored well away from light to preserve the vitamin.

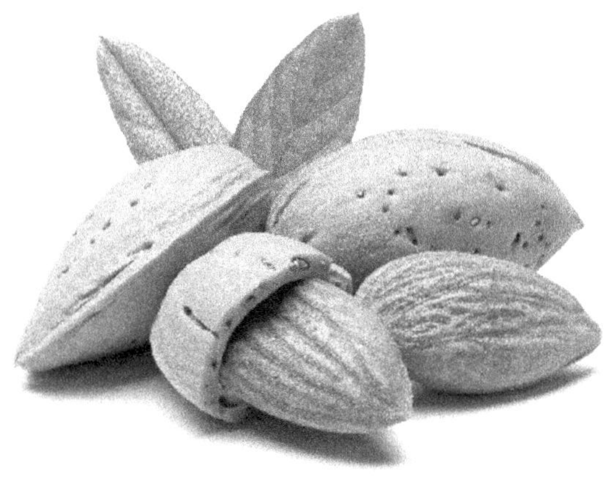

Almonds are a good source of riboflavin

We have now learned that an allergy - and a food intolerance such as that found to histamine - are underpinned by different mechanisms although symptoms may be similar.

Although intolerances and allergies offer an explanation for most of the hypersensitivity reactions such as asthma, urticaria and angioedema, it is clear that they do not explain the mystery of idiopathic angieodema. While heat and pressure angieodema are real conditions, these at least can be named; we know the cause therefore they cannot be idiopathic.

Nutritional deficiencies do need to be considered when the tests do not show up anything untoward.

Any medical specialism is still limited in what it can do; it is restricted by the powers that be who decide what can be tested for and what can be prescribed, most of which is dictated by cost. In other words, it is incomplete

It is at this point that the patient may have to separate themselves from the medical profession and undertake their own research perhaps using the medical practice as a way of obtaining tests which could work out quite expensive otherwise.

It is a failure for anyone to look forward to a lifetime of antihistamines which have some shocking side effects, often worse than the condition they were prescribed for in the first place. Antihistamines just lower the ability to fight infection leading to a lifetime of sinus problems, respiratory infections and similar.

The body is more than able to deal with the vagaries that are thrown its way provided it is given sufficient rest, exercise and nutrition.

That is what we should be aiming for.

Thank you for purchasing this book. Every time a book is purchased, a donation is made to one of the charities I am currently supporting. One such charity that has benefitted from the sale of books is The Exodus Project.

The Exodus Project

My first introduction to the far reaching impact of The Exodus Project occurred when I was travelling around Cawthorne in one of their buses, visiting gardens. A young lad was happily munching on a sandwich. He looked up briefly, pointed to the driver and said,' He's my second dad, he is,' then he returned to his sandwich without further comment.

Such remarks are often very telling and so I arranged to meet Jackie Peel and Martin Sawdon, at the charity's premises in Barnsley. They set up the Exodus Project 20 years ago. They moved into their current premises – a redundant Methodist church - in 2010.

Both Jackie and Martin have been youth workers in their church. Martin worked in housing for the homeless in addition to working in learning disabilities services in institutional settings.

The work that the Exodus Project undertakes is of paramount importance to the communities it serves. These were former mining communities which became disadvantaged after pit-closures. Currently about 400 children attend mid-week activities from Monday to Thursday inclusive. These activities include dance, drama, craft, music, sports and games. In addition, there are weekend camps, cycle treks, outward bound activities, bowling and swimming. The children are taught valuable life skills including how to cook and   bake. It is all about teaching children how to fulfil their potential and learn skills they will be able to pass onto the next generation.

The grounds, once overgrown, have been turned into   a play- and camping - ground. A miniature railway is in the process of being installed.

Martin and Jackie have developed a unique model in that The Exodus Project goes beyond dispensing services. They are keen   to build up relationships with the whole family and not just the child that attends the mid- week clubs. In addition, once children have reached the age of fourteen, they are invited to help out with the younger groups as junior volunteers. Once they reach the age of eighteen, they become adult volunteers. This   model   provides a constant supply of help from individuals   who have benefitted already from attending such groups.

The   building is large and inviting.   It is decorated with bold colours and has comfy seating. It is a real home from home; a haven for families who have been disadvantaged by the closure of the life force of its community.

Martin and Jackie have clear ideas about how they wish to develop the Exodus Project but the lottery funding which they benefitted from is no longer available. Sadly, they have had to close two of their clubs due to lack of funding.   This decision   wasn't taken lightly.   They do have two charity shops which raises some money and they obtain some funding from outside organisations for the use of their facilities. However, this is clearly not enough to keep their clubs, weekend activities   and building going to cater for the ever growing number of children who are benefitting from the work being undertaken here.   Neither does it allow for future development.

Exodus do have a Just Giving page which can be found here if you wish to help further their work https://www.justgiving.com/exodus

In addition, you can keep up with activities on their Facebook page here

https://www.facebook.com/search/top/?q=the%20exodus%20project%20barnsley&epa=SEARCH_BOX

If anyone wishes undertake an event like The Three Peaks - or run a marathon to raise funds for Exodus - then Martin or Jackie would be pleased to hear from you. This will enable their vital work in the community to continue. Contact them through their website to be found on www.exodusproject.org.uk.

Other Health Related Books by the Author

- **The Reluctant Bowel**
- **A Weighty Issue**
- **Sleep, Perchance to Dream**
- **The Journey: EDS and chronic pain**
- **The MND diet: using nutrition to slow down the progress of neurodegeneration**
- **A Necessary Sorrow**
- **Treat infection Naturally**
- **Successful Aging**
- **Taking another Road: Pain: its causes and what can be done about it**
- **Osteoarthritis and Pain**
- **A Treatment Strategy for Migraine**
- **Effective Relief for Back Pain**
- **The EDS and Hypermobility Syndrome Diet**
- **The Incontinence Diet – the latest book looking at nutritional therapy for frequency, urgency and persistent urinary tract infections**

These can be found here on the author's page

https://www.amazon.co.uk/-/e/B07BPQZ5CD

You may also be interested in the semi-autobiographical trilogy of the authors life found in these three books

- The Prejudged
- Where the Blackbird Never Sings
- A Summer's Symphony

And the author's children's books

- Fanny and Victorian Jack
- Fanny and the Gamekeeper's Cottage

www.ingramcontent.com/pod-product-compliance
Lightning Source LLC
Chambersburg PA
CBHW061354250726
48657CB00004B/1490